Purpose: The Ultimate Climax

The Guide to Finding your Purpose

Anisa Palmer

Karriem,

Thank you so much for your support. I truly appreciate you. Keep living in your Purpose King.

In Service, Anisa

Dedication

To a phenomenal woman who lived with purpose, strategically, for 38 years, my dear mother, who lost the fight to breast cancer. She wanted to publish her first book in the Spring of 1991.

Karen Palmer

April 18, 1952 – October 30, 1990

In support of Atlanta based nonprofit organization, I Will Survive, Inc. helping families battling breast cancer and health disparities across the globe to reduce generational poverty.

Support at IWillSurviveInc.org

Table of Contents

Acknowledgements

Thank you to all the incredible interns and fellows who chose to serve with I Will Survive, Inc. I wish you the best in your academic desires and careers, I hope that you find your ultimate purpose.

Thank you to all the mentees that allowed me to mentor you, I pray that you live a most fulfilled life by finding your passion to live your life with purpose. Thank you to my mentors and teachers along the way, God, Mom, Dad, Aunt Denise, Uncle Carl, Mrs. Ella Dyer, the late Ms. Lisa Dixon, Dr. Joshua Murfree, Mr. Milton Little and Mr. Roger House. Thank you to friends and family who are there with purpose.

Thank you to all the soldiers that allowed me to serve with you in the military. Thank you for entrusting me to lead you. I hope that you are living in purpose everyday.

Thank you to the IWS team, past, present and future. Thank you for your dedication and commitment to a life of serving others, a life of purpose. Thank you for allowing me to serve with you in our village, globally.

Preface

One, three, five, and seven were the ages of her girls she left behind. She was optimistic, but he knew she was not going to make it. The doctors gave her six months to live after her diagnosis of cancer. He was her husband of eight years. My father. When you know you know, they say, and dad was living proof. Dad married mom after two months. I always wondered what he did to scoop her up off her feet so quickly. Dad would say putting God first, having compatibility, and complementing one another. He remembered how beautiful she looked even after chemotherapy treatments and losing her hair. "Her skin was so radiant and the tumor had shrunk." Mom came home that day excited to feel the Caribbean sun, the ocean and the island breeze. She was even more happy to see all of her girls. Staying in Washington, D.C., she went to the National Institute of Health for treatments for a little while. Radiation was next. "I'm still down on her death date, October 30. And it still hits me on her birthday, April 18," dad said in a sad tone.

My father shared more with me about my dear mother, his late wife, in my 30s than my entire life. I wondered how he felt as a husband in those last days of her life. He shared more. I listened intently. "You were only five," he reminded me, "but you shut down. It was hard to communicate with you." Hot tears fell to my cheeks as I remembered my childhood. When one tear reached my chin, I wiped it slowly, still trying to smile. I felt her spirit near me as my father shared more. "I was there during her last breath in the hospital," my father told me. Mom jumped back on a flight, back to NIH but did not make it through radiation. It was my turn to spend time with mom during her treatments but she didn't want me to see her that way. My eldest sister spent a little time with mom while she was in chemotherapy treatments and remembered her having good days and bad days.

Good days consisted of dancing and singing in the back pews in a local Baptist Church or teaching at local schools in the United States. My sister tried to remember the hymns. Bad days consisted of throwing up due to being nauseous after all the chemicals. Smiles left photos I would take when mom left us, physically. All the images replayed in my mind. Mom was raised Catholic after being adopted. Dad was baptized as a Baptist and, as adults, they both explored Islam. Mom's mother had a Polish background and her father had served in the military. Mom was fluent in Spanish, Swahili, English, Arabic and a few other African languages. She was a global citizen.

"Mom made every day special, even when she was sick." My sister recalled, walking down the street and seeing a snake for the first time while visiting mom in treatments on the mainland. The snake had a pale yellowish complexion and was large to a six-year-old, months shy of turning seven. We did not have snakes on the island. Mongooses were imported to rid the snakes during the African Diaspora. "Mom made me unafraid." She sat up, remembered, and said smiling from ear to ear, "mom always made everything okay. I became fearless with mom and touched the snake."

Everything changed for our family in February of 1990 when mom felt pain in her breast. In March, it was confirmed: mom was diagnosed with the worst form of aggressive breast cancer. The biopsy came back positive for Infectious Carcinoma, Stage IV. It had not even been a year since mom had given birth to her last daughter, her fifth child, Miriam, righteously named after Miriam Makeba from South Africa. Mom prayed for girls after her son, and, well... to say she was happy would be an understatement.

An Open Letter to Mom

Dear Mom,

You are my hero! I love you so much! Thank you for planting the seeds. Thank you for giving me a piece of peace. Thank you for sticking your finger down my throat to make me throw up that penny I had accidentally swallowed. You saved my life. Thank you for nurturing me. Thank you for my name. Thank you for making the most amazing meals. I was never hungry after you cooked and my stomach was always satisfied. Thank you for making birthdays special, I try to ensure I make others feel special as well on their birthdays. Thank you for singing to me, your beautiful voice. Playing the piano, all the instruments.

I love music because of you. Thank you for art. My escape at my darkest moments in life. I was in a center for abused teens and I used art to help me heal. Voluminous seeds you planted. They bloomed when they needed to, you prepared me to allow myself to heal. I made lemonade with lemons.

Thank you for dancing and keeping the culture alive. Dancing makes me feel like you are guiding me onto the dance floor even when I do not have a partner to dance with. Thank you for all of your poems, your flow is incomparable. All of your children are poets and we have all recited to each other or in poetry spots all across the globe. Your oldest daughter is going to publish her first cookbook soon; you are her inspiration. My sisters are married to great men, they treat them with respect and provide through love. They complement them and are compatible with them. They always keep God first. Your grandchildren are smart and full of energy. They know about you! One did a school project about you and breast cancer. He lives in Florida. Your son is learning how to be a great father. We always check on him as you would have wanted. We have so much love for each other - you poured so much into us. We are good people, we have great values, manners, and are respectable human beings. Mom, thank you for providing a village, globally. I have met extraordinary people around the world that love you. They say nothing but positive things about the woman you were. I am so proud to be your daughter. Your birthday is the official "I Will Survive" day in the city of Doraville, right outside of Atlanta, Georgia. I keep in touch with many of your friends. The Williams family still keep our family in prayers, a true joy to hang with them in 2009. Mama ChinzeRa is now a professor at the University of the Virgin Islands and the children have grown up to be incredible human beings. Your dear friend, Adjoa, is still dancing and singing all over the islands. Elisa McKay, I saw for the first time since your death. She is incredible, doing and teaching yoga still in her 80's and full of so much life. I met up with her when I went home in the summer of 2018. We laughed and hugged each other, smiled, and laughed some more. We shared a meal in Christiansted at Franks new restaurant, BES Craft Cocktail Lounge. Everything was delicious, you would have loved it. We ordered vegan mushroom burgers and the saltfish tostones were additional for me. The best! Craving some now actually. The salt fish wasn't too salty and the tostones were made to perfection. They had the perfect crisp to them.

Thank you for meeting my dad and allowing him to sweep you off your feet in two months! Thank you for carrying me for 9 months and feeding your body nourishment so I was born a healthy baby. Thank you for being my teacher, literally and figuratively. Having the children in our home from the neighborhood taught me early, the importance of education. Amongst all your children, we hold several degrees and keep on seeking the knowledge inside and outside the classroom. Undergrad at Georgia State University, I know you sent me Dr. Holmes. She was the absolute best. I chose to minor in theatre because of you. Thank you for introducing me to acting and plays. You gave countless children a positive outlet in Lew Muckle Elementary School with theatre down the street from our home in our neighborhood, Sion Farm.

I know you were there, spiritually, with my first car accident, my first financial loss, my first heartbreak, my first success. Thank you for helping me get my credit together to buy my first house. And a special thank you for helping me pick it out. Upon closing, my real estate agent donated his earnings to my favorite charity, I know that was you. Thank you!

My Angel! Thank you for being there for the awards, the speeches, the accolades, and most importantly... the hardest moments of my life. You helped me survive the rough days and find my purpose. Thank you for giving me the courage to share this story to help someone else in their journey to purpose.

I Love You Always and I hope to make you proud!

Your Daughter,

Anisa

A Piece of Peace by Karen Palmer

I lived a full life - full of happiness!
A learned a lot
A lot about hurt and misery.
As a child I got away with murder
And grew up killing myself.
"Stop," said I, "I must seek refuge."
And so I inscape into the world for comfort.
I became frightened.
There you were.
Aid has never meant much –
Just three letters.
But now those three letters mean something.
A for acceptance
I for intelligence
D for discreteness – you!
You aided me and I thank you.
I thank you for giving me myself.

To help was to hinder
To hinder was to love.
Hate was to love –
Happiness was loneliness.
Loneliness was misery.
You helped me see the light.
Life was darkness but has become the key
To love and peace. Peace of mind.
You are always welcomed.

From you I got a piece of peace.

I give you this poem in exercise of the freedom You helped me
to find! *Dedicated to Dr. Mary Donaldson on January 9, 1971.*

"Positive is How I Live."

~ Virgin Islands motto

Chapter **1**

Affirmations: Positive is How I Live

Imagine if we could breathe together. Imagine if I could inhale and you, exhale. Human beings tend to take destructive lifestyles to cover the pain. What if you could turn that pain into purpose? Why let our anger become the devil's remote control? Allow me to help as we move through these chapters together.

It took many years to be able to talk about my mom without crying. Even so, tears have already fallen on the page in front of me. There's just so much. So much to tell. My strength to continue comes from the fact that somebody needs to hear my story, not so they can get to know me better, but so they can get to know themselves. Someone reading this needs to see the purpose buried beneath their pain.

Pain is like a mysterious stranger. It can be hard to understand because you don't know when you'll see it again. It can be diabolical because it seems to know the worst time to visit you. And as if that weren't enough, the deepest pain doesn't have a voice. We cry, but tears can't come close to expressing certain losses in our life. But I'm going to try my best. Hopefully, my words will connect to experiences deep down. Experiences that have shaped how we see the world and everyone in it.

I've learned there is no situation beyond the reach of God's healing hand. Nothing can happen to us that can destroy the purpose God has for our lives. There is a reason we are here. There is a reason you are reading this right now. This is my story. I really hope, one day, to hear yours.

I was just a little girl when breast cancer took my mother. I was only five. Right when I was learning about life, the most important one of all had been taken from me. The pain from such a loss doesn't care about how young you are.

The pain doesn't care that this is the time when you should be playing with toys and going to birthday parties. Pain doesn't care, but God does.

My mother's death changed everything for me. The sun dimmed a little. Even midnight darkened. The common, mundane things you may have taken for granted now have new meaning. Even days of the week are different. Fridays became the best day of the week for a good reason. In elementary school we went across the street to the beach every Friday. The ocean became an escape. The way it sounds. The way it feels. Nature helped me reconnect in a strangely peaceful way.

I still remember a lot from that period in my life. I remember little things, like Mom's favorite color - purple. Royal purple of the Queens and Kings in the magnificent continent of Africa. Purple, also the color of prevention in the health world. Mom also loved green. Lush green of Mother Nature. She smelled of the beautiful essence of the Blue Nile that came in the form of an essential oil. It was her favorite. I remember all of this. She loved the beach. Maybe that is why I also love it to this day. The deep, succulent blue you see after you pass the aquamarine blue in the shallow areas. There is a place in life, a deeper place you can only see after you rid yourself of shallow things, shallow people, shallow ideas, shallow ambitions. A deeper place where our thinking is bathed in understanding. In all of our lives, there is a place called deeper blue.

Mom used to sit next to the water all day sometimes. I would sit next to her playing in the waves. I remember the first time I tasted the sand. She laughed as I tasted the grittiness in my teeth. With mom, I was free. I felt whole. I wish I could hear her call my name once more.

Let me ask you, what is your earliest memory of experiencing love and acceptance from someone in your life? Do you remember the first positive comment someone said to you? Words that made you feel confident about yourself. Was it your mom, your brother, your teacher or mentor? Who first gave you an insight into who you could be one day? While you consider this question, let me tell you a little more by way of background.

I was born and raised in the Virgin Islands, on St. Croix. We were purchased by the United States from the Danish in 1917 for $25 million. If you ask me, they got us for really cheap. If you study our history, you'll see we have been under the rule of Spain, France, England and Denmark. Our motto growing up has stayed with me even till this day: 'positive is how I live.'

The Virgin Islands, once called the Danish West Indies, does not consist of secret islands holding a plethora of gorgeous virgins to your liking. It does, however, consist of three islands called St. Thomas, St. John, and St. Croix (en español - Santa Cruz). People from St. Croix are identified as Cruzan. Some may be familiar with our famous Cruzan Rum or visited the island. St. Croix is 82 square miles around and the largest of the three islands. Every school I attended had a beach within close proximity so I really could say "right near de beach" when someone asked me where I went to school.

Leaving the islands in my teenage years, I swam across the Atlantic Ocean and began my journey on new soils to create a new life. I wanted to travel the world, but culture shock cut me short. After my mother passed away, my brother moved to the United States and I was right behind him. In the states, I learned that I came from a "broken family" and that island folks have no cars or houses. I really did not swim across the ocean, by the way. I also learned that island folks seem to smoke marijuana and listen to Bob Marley. Or, at least that's what the stereotype said. The stereotypes were just horrible.

Years later while living in the states, I found that I was still grieving over my mother. I was older, more mature, but in many ways, I was still that five-year-old little girl wondering where her mother went. Kate Atwood, a grief expert in Atlanta, reminded me that it is okay to grieve a loved one. There is no expiration date or artificial timeline you have to obey. Kate founded Kate's Club, which helps youths dealing with loss. This became her passion after losing her mother to breast cancer. We had a lot in common. I had the privilege of volunteering with her organization in partnership with the Junior League of Atlanta.

I smile when remembering something Mom used to say. 'Be a good person.' If I heard this once, I heard it a thousand times. This was her daily melody. It would be years before I understood why. Today, I realize she was planting a seed for a time when she wouldn't be around. Times when I would need a mature perspective. Times when I may be confused about what to do. Times when I would need a principle I could depend on. It is a simple statement, yet profound in its application, 'be a good person.' The saying itself solves many problems.

Many years after moving to the US, I went back home to to visit the islands. Of course, when it was time to return to the US, I wanted to bring back mementos. I had coconuts, sand, a little jar of salt water from the beach, and fresh exotic fruit in my luggage... only to be taken away from me in Customs. The US has brought me a mixed bag of experiences. My heart was broken for the first time at the tender age of 18 years. On the other hand, I went into the import and export business here and made my first million before the age of 21. However, cash did not rule everything around me. Smile.

I served in the Armed Forces for four years, completing two tours in Iraq during Operation Iraqi Freedom. I survived war. I made it back from Iraq. Some of my battle buddies did not. Survival is an interesting word - I call it that because, contrary to the cliché, the strongest don't always survive. Sometimes the wounded do. Sometimes the "weak" do. Sometimes the grieving does.

I've survived many things. Growing up, it was a task to just survive the weather. I can remember having a wind specialist walking through to ensure we allowed the harsh winds to pass through without picking up our Virgin Islands home in Sion Farm from its very foundation. In the Virgin Islands, we lost many lives to Hurricane Hugo. I remember as if it were yesterday.

Our neighbor's roof had been torn off completely. Their roof ended up down the street in a shopping center. Hugo destroyed so much. Mom survived Hugo, but then again, she was a survivor by nature. She survived trauma as an adopted child, dealt with an identity crisis as well as a divorce, more than once. I want to know a little about you, yes, you the reader. What have you survived? Put a check next to your subject of survival below.

Rape
War
Flood
Fire

Divorce

Bullying

Hurricanes

Broken Heart

Start-up of a Business

Loss of a Business

Gossip

Tornado

Breast Cancer or other

Domestic Violence

Homelessness

Abuse

Loss of a Loved One

Loss of Employment

Sexual Harassment

Foreclosure

Bankruptcy

Embarrassment

Illness/Disease

Adoption

Human Trafficking

Prison

Hate Crime

Murder of a Loved One

Toxic Masculinity

Gun Violence

I checked off quite a few things from this list. Did reading the list take you back? Look at where you are now. Envision where you want to be in the future. How can you get there? How can we get there together?

When my mother was diagnosed, I had no idea how much the disease would shape my life. Her sickness gave me purpose, gave me a mission that would eventually affect the lives of many. I founded *I Will Survive*, Incorporated, a 501 (c) (3) with a mission to provide prevention education, economic support, and health and wellness services to those at higher risk and those affected by breast cancer. Founded in 2010 and based out of Atlanta, Georgia, the organization plans to branch out to the Caribbean, South America, and Africa.

Do me a favor and like the organization on Facebook, and follow on Instagram @IWillSurviveInc. I'll wait... all done? Great! Thank you for your support. Now back to the story.

Through my creator, and yes, through the trial He sent my way, I found my purpose. There are times when we believe trials come from the enemy, but have you ever considered that your trial may have come from God? What do you do when tribulation, and persecution is God-ordained. How do you handle hell that comes from heaven?

My mother was my ultimate foundation after God. She was a true woman of virtue. Everything about her captivated me in many ways. Just to feel her touch brought me peace. Her eyes held the secrets of a successful life, a life of true happiness. Mom's skin was soft. Her smile, her laugh was healing to the soul. She was my everything.

If you visited the Virgin Islands back in those days you would have noticed how all of the children in the community were drawn to my mom. To hear her beautiful voice singing and playing piano, or dancing and singing would do my spirit good right now. These were my thoughts with tears in my eyes at 12 years old. God please let me squeeze mom once more. Kiss one more time. Read me a bedtime story and tuck me in. Breast cancer became my enemy even though she left with no more pain. She died peacefully. Her only worry was for her children. She prayed we would be okay. I was not okay. A piece of me died when she left physically. I wondered that very moment, could I ever be whole again? My first love was my mother. Her lips were pink and full. Her hair was dark with waves that fell down to her back until chemotherapy released the roots. Her skin was reluctant to pick up the sun beams. She was beyond beautiful and the happiest woman in the world in its simplicity. That was how she wanted to be remembered. She often told them not to worry about her and not to cry for her. I cried for hours. Sometimes I cried for many days at a time.

Breast cancer has a personality, a face, an attitude and I hated all of it. The smell, the look, the touch, the meaning, the month, October. I hated, the National Breast Cancer Awareness Month, the pink ribbons, the pink everywhere, and painting it pretty. What is pretty about breast cancer? People wear it almost like it's a holiday.

The way it sounded rolling off a doctor's tongue telling someone else, "you have breast cancer." The tumor that became malignant. In the beginning, I was a neophyte to breast cancer. It used to have no meaning. Not even a thought. Then all of a sudden, it devoured my days and nights with a hunger beyond imagination. You see, I woke up and it would already be on my mind. It controlled my life. In the early days, I quickly realized that breast cancer was more than a disease. It was a monstrous plague that took out nations and civilizations. It snuck up on people that were needed in the world. As much as some of us want to believe that everyone needs someone, there are actually some people that exist that no one needs and if they died tomorrow, many will not care. Yes, that may seem cruel, but it is true. The serial rapists in the world, mass murderers; who needed them anyway?

People like my mother were needed and perhaps still needed by many. She was a leader, and many were lost without her. Homes fell apart, as well as neighborhoods and nations. I learned that a house did not make a home from Luther Vandross, and from my own home that fell into a nonexistent state when breast cancer took my dear mother. I lived in many houses over the course of my life and thought I would never be able to have a home again. My mother not only made a home, she was home.

Steps to finding purpose in your life.

1. What are some things you overcame or survived?

_____

_____

_____

_____

_____

_____

_____

2. What brings you the most joy, legally?

_____

_____

_____

_____

_____

"The two most important days in your life are the day you are born and the day you find out why." ~ Mark Twain

Chapter **2**

Journey to Purpose

I passed the fastest kid in school, Kevin. I was surely going to the Olympics after I joined the track team. My sister still reminds me that I could have been a champion in my adult years. I was barely 12 years old then. My father did not allow me to play sports in any extracurricular activities even though my coach, our Physical Education teacher wanted me to. I was lucky I was even in private school.

I stared at the crack made by Hurricane Hugo in the house that day. If mom was alive, I thought, I would be on the track team. My grades were terrible. I only excelled in Art and P.E. Dad said, "focus on your grades." My rebuttal was, "my grades would be better if I could join the team." He wasn't buying it. Dad ended up getting hit by a drunk driver riding his Harley Davidson motorcycle to work in my preteen years and is still in a wheelchair to this day. I missed riding on the back of the bike with dad, speeding past all the pain.

I grew up a tomboy in the Virgin Islands. I played international futbol (soccer) and American football as told from the movie, The Waterboy (1998), with American actor, comedian, screenwriter, and film producer, Adam Sandler. I also played baseball, softball, volleyball, basketball, kickball, and dodgeball. I climbed trees and had nasty pus gushing out my kneecaps when I fell. I did not wear skirts or dresses when I started to dress myself as a little girl. I burped out loud and had farting contests. I won a few. Oh, and I hated pink.

Ironically, pink loved me. Pink has now grown to have a love/hate relationship with me. I hate that we are gendered at birth, girls to wear pink and play with Barbie dolls and boys to wear blue and fight and never cry. I still hate, dislike, that some men who get breast cancer have a fear of speaking about it publicly because of the color pink and its association with women's breasts. A shade of blue is supposed to be used for male breast cancer, do you ever see that ribbon? No one has.

On the other hand, I like pink because the color has become a stance for support, a call to action to survive, a proclamation to fight, pride of survival, unity for communities, and a band bridging families, coworkers, and friends together for support of loved ones. It's a complicated relationship when what stands for support also stands for pain.

I do like pink because an amazing volunteer created my logo for my nonprofit organization. He came down from Boston and was looking for a job after graduating from college. Joel Premier is his name. Originally from Sierra Leone, he did an amazing job of the logo. I am not being biased - you should have seen it before. I like pink enough to want to see it more than just in the month of October. Now, you're probably thinking, 'Anisa is confused. Does she like or hate pink?!' Well, I want people to care about breast cancer during the other eleven months of the year, volunteer to help someone survive not only when there is pink glitter, and I don't want people to donate just because American football athletes are decked out in pink gear.

Pink... I dislike you, but I like you and I hope we all will survive even when pink or peach (the original color: see documentary Pink Ribbons, Inc., 2011) aren't cheering us on. There is a growing population of breast cancer survivors in general, but why is the mortality rate for minority women, when it comes to breast cancer, highest compared to the majority, Caucasian women of non-Jewish descent? The minority is all the rest of the women with a high focus on African descended and women of Jewish descent. These two populations have the highest prevalence of BRCA 1 and BRCA 2 gene or the breast cancer genes. Famous actress and humanitarian, Angelina Jolie, got her BRCA gene test in 2013. Since then, it has become a hugely controversial issue. Some women have decided to take their personal approach to preventive care against breast cancer after finding positive results for the breast cancer gene. Some have taken the approach of removing their breast tissue and replacing them with breast implants. Many women feel breasts reflect womanhood and, without them, they feel less of a woman.

Now, Breast Implant Illness is coming to light as more and more women suffer from the side effects of having implants. Others have chosen to change their lifestyles by drastically decreasing the intake of certain foods and increasing the amounts of other cancer fighting foods as well as removing toxins in their life. Toxins, sometimes even in the form of people. The only things more damaging than eating unhealthy food, is being around unhealthy people, unhealthy opinions, and a lack of support that can make you doubt your own abilities. I will touch on this in more detail in chapter three.

I wanted the test done. I needed the cancer test, but my insurance company had other opinions. It is interesting how you sometimes have to fight for what's right, but this time, I was ready to fight! I fought my own health insurance to get the

BRCA gene test done. I was back on the battlefield. A battle I did not want to be in. It was me against the healthcare system or 'sick care system' of the United States of America. I had no one on my side but stood tall and strong ready for whatever would come my way. I was told that I needed to have two people who passed away prior to be given this test in 2013. Since my dear mother was adopted, how was there a way to find out if more than two had passed away already and the most important question... why wait for more to die?

My case was finally won and I began my genetic counselling before testing. I had many sleepless nights worried about if I had the gene or not, and what it would mean to be a daughter who lost her mother to breast cancer, as a sister who had more sisters, as a woman in leadership with a breast cancer organization. "1 in 8 women will be diagnosed with breast cancer in her lifetime," according to the American Cancer Society and the Center for Disease Control and Prevention. About 1 in 1000 men will be diagnosed with breast cancer in their lifetime. Yes, men can get breast cancer too.

Men have breast tissue. I can tell you from my experience, sometimes you have to fight for what's right. If there is something in your life you want and you need, do not give up. Do not allow someone to convince you to let go. Fight, fight, fight. Rest if you must, but get up to fight again.

I remember sitting in a window comfort seat on a Delta flight watching the sunset. It was a beautiful view on an MD-88 aircraft. Orange, red, and a hint of pink, of course. I was on my way to New York to visit my long-time friend whom I hadn't seen in a while. It was also very close to my birthday and I had created a life I did not need a vacation from, my journey through purpose. My friend was also a massage therapist and created outstanding health products that I needed to purchase, as an avid supporter of small, minority-owned businesses.

While on the aircraft, I began to think about all the great things I had accomplished thus far. I also thought about all the things I still needed to accomplish without going into the erroneous zones of worry and guilt that the late Wayne W. Dyer explains. The past can sabotage our future because the future needs our attention. As long as the past has us thinking about our past, our future will starve to death.

For me, my past can be difficult to forget. I was raped. I was 17 years old, I was still new to the United States and just beginning college on a merit program to start higher education early. I was distraught. I felt violated and disgusted. I dropped out of college. I could not face my rapist. If I moved on to live my life in worry of the potential next person that could rape me, how on earth could I live my life for the now? Loving my life for the present means enjoying every moment. People had always asked me if I had regret joining the military. I would always tell them "no" without hesitation. Why? In life we learn to make lemonade with the lemons. Enjoy the good, the bad, and the ugly. It made me the person I am today. I took the lemons life threw at me, did a Caribbean wine to twist all the juices, added a little sugar cane in the raw, so I would not be too sour about it, and finished with a smile on it.

———

I oftentimes share with breast cancer survivors through my nonprofit organization that God only gives the strongest battles to the strongest soldiers. This is true, but sometimes God simply selects a person and places emotional protection around them. Sometimes you're just chosen. My mother was both tough and chosen. After giving birth to five unique children, she was diagnosed with stage IV invasive breast cancer. Because she lost the battle to breast cancer does not mean she lost the war. She left the earth smiling knowing that her children would go on to accomplish great things. She did not have any guilt or worry which allowed her to enjoy the moments cherishing her children while she was still on earth. She smiled daily through the pain of chemotherapy and often times questioned her friends for crying when they came to visit her. "If I am not crying, why are you?" she would ask them.

During her last breath, when the malignant tumor had metastasized to her lungs, she was still smiling. But I cried knowing that mommy would not be there anymore. As a child, my grieving turned to fear and worry. My little sister held all the guilt and thought that if she were never born, mommy would still be alive. She finally let that guilt out at the tender age of 21, when I took her to visit mom's gravesite.

Everyone grieves differently. Another good friend of mine and mentor, Gail, is a grieving coach in Florida. She had shared some wisdom with me on this topic and mentioned that my grieving process has still continued in the work I do with my nonprofit organization, part of my purpose. She explained to me that I now carry my mother as a mother carries a child in their womb. I thought that was so deep. Gail, slightly older and wiser than myself, allowed me to really analyze myself further with her wisdom. My grieving process has given me strength rather than destroying me. Because of this, one of my goals in life has been to help others do the same with regards to living a positive purposeful life through coaching.

Grieving steps can also be used in relationships when they are on the verge of being over. Why be sad about it? Enjoying each moment means being happy about the good, the bad, and the ugly. In relationships, even if he or she did you wrong, find moments when you learned something new about yourself. You think you may hate him or her, but why allow them to have that much control over your emotions? You are in charge of your feelings. Live for the present. Find happy moments several times throughout your day. Find reasons to smile and share them. You may just make someone else's day as well while sharing that beautiful smile. So, go ahead and smile, as Instagram Influencer @Mr_Hotspot reminds us all, "like that."

To start, write down some positive affirmations and post them by your mirror in your bathroom when you brush your teeth in the morning. If you do not brush your teeth in the morning, we need not worry, as Dr. Dyer would suggest; you have some serious hygiene issues that can only be resolved by acting now. If you are in Atlanta, make an appointment with my dentist today, Dr. Freemont with Freemont Dental, and let them know I referred you. Clean teeth help make you happy.

If you travel often, take your positive affirmations with you and leave the paper on your nightstand in your hotel or Airbnb so you can say them as soon as you rise. I recently heard a young 6-year-old girl recite her positive affirmations in front of an audience of women entrepreneurs next to her mother, who went from being an inmate in prison to an inspiration to several youths. I was receiving the Legacy Award with the *I Am Awards* in Atlanta, Georgia, and Desiree Lee moved the audience with her story of being an inmate. I was moved even more by listening to her young daughter share her positive affirmations. If she can do it, I know you can.

This leads us into our principles to living your life with purpose. No matter what horrific moments you have encountered, you are a survivor. You overcame. You are a winner. Even if you do not win all the battles, you can win the war. The Anisa Palmer Principles can be incorporated into your life to reduce stress and live your life with purpose with purpose. Once you have them down, you will begin to realize that you also let go of worry, guilt, fear and boosted your health and confidence. The following chapters will break these principles down so you can see how living your life with purpose is vital for a healthy, quality life.

In Your Journey to Purpose.

1. What can you do for someone else who have felt the pain you have felt?

_____

_____

_____

_____

_____

_____

_____

_____

2. How could helping someone else with empathy help you too?

_____

_____

_____

_____

_____

"Don't get caught up in the life you are living, get caught up to live your life with purpose." ~ Anisa Palmer

Chapter 3

Strategize to the Climax

Living a life of purpose helps you reach the ultimate climax. Want to climax every day? Who doesn't! In this chapter you will learn:

1. Ways to live your life with purpose to reach climax
2. How passion feeds purpose to reach a daily climatic lifestyle
3. What to do to become inspired to take purposeful action
4. How to add life to your years = more climactic moments

It was my second deployment in Iraq when I saw a rose. My mother's nickname was Rose; it was a mirage of my mother. It finally hit me. Mom looked as beautiful as I could remember. I was once living to die from grief, but now I'm dying to live from purpose. My mission had been assigned and accepted from the Most High. I thought I would retire in the military with 25 years at least to reach the rank of Major

General. I was inspired by women like Admiral Michelle

Howard in the Navy, General Janet Wolfbarger in the Air

Force, and General Ann Dunwoody in the Army. General

Dunwoody commanded at the same duty station I was at, Fort

Bragg, North Carolina, the home of the 82nd Airborne Division

and she was the first woman to serve as a general on this base.

I knew when I went to my first competition board for

early promotion after my second deployment in Iraq, that I

would become an author, as I wrote it in my biography then. I

did not know that I would not be in the military when I

published my first book, but I am grateful for every journey

and proud to say that my soldiers looked up to me and

respected me as a woman, a leader, and a soldier. I am

honored to have served and I still carry the Army values with

me daily. I would not trade anything in the world for my

service. I serve now in various other forms of purpose. My

mother's spirit and strength were with me through every

mission and every moment and I will forever dedicate my life

to her as I live with purpose. The Army gave me wings, but

God gave them to me first. Airborne! For all my fellow maroon berets.

Purposeful action occurs when we strategically plan after a revelation. A large poster of T.D. Jakes quotes, "If you can't figure out your purpose, figure out your passion. For your passion will lead you right into your purpose." It is displayed in my nonprofit organization office as a constant reminder of my purpose journey. I always had a passion for helping others. It could be tied to my zodiac sign or simply my desire to serve. I was eager to join the military to serve not knowing anything about the military itself. I mistakenly thought it was similar to the Peace Corps. Ignorance may not always be bliss, or was it?

In Chapter One, I shared how we all survive something. I used to be afraid of heights. While in the military, I was offered to go to any duty station after completing some training at Fort Lee, Virginia. I first chose Italy, not knowing that I would enjoy it better outside of the military in 2014. I then chose Djibouti, located in the Horn of Africa. I got a little more specific, as I really wanted to go to Africa, but my leaders again encouraged me to pick someplace in the United States of America. I asked important questions as I was still new to the mainland and have not been to many states at all. I knew the right questions to ask without reading *Good Leaders Ask Great Questions* by John Maxwell. After gathering all the information that I needed, I chose Fort Bragg, North Carolina to become a Paratrooper. Yes, the person who didn't like heights was going to be a paratrooper!

I was able to pick my next duty station because I completed training in the top of my class. They asked me to stay to compete in the Audie Murphy Board. I turned down the prestigious competitive board to go on to complete my next mission, purpose. The mission that would change my life and reveal my purpose to me was approaching fast. I completed Airborne School at Fort Benning, which straddled the Alabama - Georgia border. I then went back to Fort Bragg to soon deploy on my first overseas tour in support of Operation Iraqi Freedom in 2008. I no longer had a fear of heights and reached my first climactic moment while jumping from a C-130 Hercules aircraft, purpose.

Putting on the Army uniform helped me see a leader in the mirror everyday while serving in the military. I needed to see that leader to believe in myself to accomplish my ultimate mission, or reach the ultimate climax. Becoming more than the uniform was the joy in the stepping stone leading up to my ultimate purpose. The passion of serving others was feeding my purpose to start a nonprofit organization to help families battling breast cancer in disadvantaged populations. I was not ready until I had overcome all the adversities, trials and tribulations, lemons and bad apples.

When you live your life with purpose, you wake up smiling every day with a positive attitude. When you smile every day and laugh, you release positive endorphins. There has been a great increase of Laughter Yoga Instructors around the globe. We all need more laughter in our lives. We need those smiles, climactic moments. We find them when we are living our lives purposefully. It takes more muscles to frown than laugh, and fascinating research confirms satisfaction in life and longevity is based on smiling. If you are not happy with your smile, it is okay, you can see my dentist, mentioned earlier.

When we think of climactic moments that make us happiest, some have sexual memories or desires, in the past or future. How about thinking of the present, it is a gift after all! The things that make us most fulfilled, give us the most passion, which leads us straight to our purpose.

If you are an alpha, beta, or omega personality type (type A personality) and you are also a giver, you have to be careful not to lose yourself in the service of others. Find balance. Getting burned out helping people and putting yourself last doesn't help anybody. Health is our greatest wealth. Nonprofit leaders, mothers, teachers, service industry professionals along with type A personalities ... listen clearly!

Are you the type that takes client calls on your direct line at 11:00pm at night? Are you the one that always buys the extra school supplies when your classroom does not have them? Are you also sitting on several boards, working another job or two, and still leading ministry groups or other groups? You need balance.

Balance is the only way to make it all work, long-term. Relationships, whether they are friendships or not, suffer when one gives and the other always takes. I am living proof. Even if the other individual feels as though they are giving something, you may not even be receiving it if what they are giving is not your love language.

You have to be able to know how or what to give in friendships, relationships, marriages to make them work. In business, if your team needs awards to show they are appreciated, then awards need to be given. If your team needs free lunch a few times throughout the year or once a week, do it! Find a way. When you invest in the team, the friendship, the relationship, the marriage... it has the ability to last an eternity or just as long as it needs to last. God's plan, not ours. Reason, season or lifetime. Not all things are meant for eternity.

In our monthly team meetings at the office for the charity, my goal was to understand the type of dynamic, inclusive, diverse team we had, in order to cater to each of their needs so they could be as productive as possible. In addition, we all were able to boost employee morale simultaneously.

I remember when one of my directors of a department sent me a video about business and how not everyone on the team is meant to stay. This director understood the importance of team players and what it took to have a strong team. Prior to him joining our team, he built successful teams with various Fortune 500 companies and went on to build his own business. He built it to be so great that someone wanted to buy it. Chris was a great leader on our team to the charity.

I learned that I did not want to be the smartest person on my team, so I was doing everything alone. That took the passion out of my purpose. Hire people that add value to the team, to the business, for transformational or transactional leadership. When a team player no longer wants to play on the team, get rid of them fast. They have the potential to cause disruption in your organizational culture. If you are a first-time leader, identify who these people are. Stay woke, even if it is not your business that you started yourself.

> "When we have potential in our business and it does not realize its true value, you have to let it go. Sometimes someone with less potential can provide better value because of their effort. Potential is nothing without effort." – *Chris Williams*, Founder, Elite Web Professionals & Marketing Director, I Will Survive, Inc.

I wholeheartedly believe that our overall purpose does not change. Goals change. Vision changes. Mission changes.

Passion changes. My purpose was with me all along. A new passion came to serve in a new way, I was already serving.

I love when we wore name badges at a TED Talks event with our purpose written under our name. Some had theirs blank, when able to fill it out when registering for the event. They were still trying to identify what their purpose was. Strategically, you can find it, by always listening to your passion and understanding how passions come together, like a puzzle. How do all the passions fit, if you have more than one?

A musician can may one day no longer have a passion to play the flute, but still love the way music moves people. A joy to tickle the ear drums with tight beats, incredible purpose. I applaud musicians and thank them for sharing their gifts with us.

A teacher may one day no longer have a passion to teach 1st graders, but still love teaching and the positive impact they have on students. They could enjoy high school students more. When purpose hits, it feels so good, the ultimate climax!

When these shifts occur in life, it can be disruptive, a shift of passion in your purpose. For example, in a marriage, you and your spouse work in your respective fields. You are a medical doctor and your spouse, an engineer. One day someone wakes up and has a change of calling, passion in purpose. Or purpose never fulfilled and finally listening to the calling they once ignored. Now, they want to be a spiritual leader, a calling they feel from their creator. How do you support your spouse in this new space?

Does faith pull you through? Household income changes, the number one reason for divorce? Does infidelity occur, someone steps out because they feel betrayed? Children are impacted. The sooner you find your purpose, the better your life and the lives of those around you.

The below are steps to reaching climax, the ultimate purpose, in your life. It helps to know what brings you joy and what does not.

1. List some of your passions in life:

_____

_____

_____

_____

_____

_____

2. List things that do not move you at all:

_____

_____

_____

_____

_____

"Life is 10% what happens to you and 90% how you react to it."

~ Charles R. Swindoll

Chapter **4**

Attitude: Put A Smile on It

Pictures without smiles. My childhood had many.
I received one that I had never seen before from my uncle and
aunt in my late 20's and saw a baby picture of myself for the
first time. I was smiling. I was happy. Mom must have taken
that photo.

If you're happy then you should have put a smile on it.
Beyoncé remake! Attitude is everything. I walked into the front
office for my nonprofit organization and listened to a team
member answer the phone in a very sad tone. He explained he
was happy after the phone call, or at least he thought he was.

We can feel a frown through the phone - same with
anger, disappointment, frustration. I had someone tell me
once, in my early teenage years that she knew when I was on

my menstrual cycle. A few years later, I concentrated on being the nicest person with the most upbeat attitude when my cycle was on. It helped me during my military training when rough days came as I certainly did not feel like conducting inventory on millions of dollars' worth of equipment in Supply Chain Management in the cold rainy weather. I had to get it done and no one would know how I truly felt about it because of the smile that was planted on my face.

I wanted to become an Army Ranger when women were not allowed to. I became frustrated inside, discussing the importance of going to Ranger School to my Commander in order to help boost my career, since I thought I would stay in the military to become a General. I wore a smile outside and carried out my duties as assigned, not knowing that God had another plan for me, and it was not becoming an Army Ranger or a General, or even completing the Audie Murphy Board. All those titles didn't matter once my purpose was revealed to me but I needed the positive attitude to get to each climactic moment in order to reach the ultimate climax.

I almost did not graduate Basic Combat Training or boot camp when I first served in the Armed Forces. I suffered from pneumonia and hypothermia - yes, at the same damn time! I was in the Emergency Room for pneumonia after training in the winter months of South Carolina, Fort Jackson. My body had not fully adjusted to the cold weather yet. My Caribbean blood was still flowing through my internal dimensions. My Drill Sergeant knew of my leadership potential before I saw it in myself. He made me Platoon Leader and I felt like I had let my platoon down by being admitted into the ER. I came back stronger than ever and learned some valuable lessons. There will be times when we have to rest, especially in our purpose. Listen to our bodies so we can come back even stronger and smile even wider. After all, health is our greatest wealth!

I told the incredible intern in my office that day that it is okay to have a bad day. Go home and handle what you need to handle and come back tomorrow stronger than ever to accomplish the mission. The intern was able to handle the situation and come back a new person the next day. The intern later held a leadership position in the organization. Leaders or not, self-care matters!

We have to take care of ourselves before we can truly take care of anyone else. There is a reason we must put the oxygen mask on ourselves first in the airplane before helping someone else place his or her oxygen mask on.

"If you don't like something, change it. If you can't change it, change your attitude," Maya Angelou reminds us. Our attitude can block our blessings, have doors shut on us, or even have us miss our purpose being revealed to us. We must keep our eyes open (stay woke) and strategically be ready. How can we be ready for something we do not even know? What will it look like? When will it come?

We have to be careful who we marry as well when it comes to purpose. We have to understand commitment, compatibility, compassion, and compromise. Former First Lady Michelle Obama wrote *Becoming*, sharing the woman she became to support her husband through his purpose of becoming the first African American President in the United States for not one, but two terms. Eight years of her life. His purpose became her purpose although she did not ever want to work in politics. His passion became her passion in love, but she still had to live for herself too. Eight years of their life. A team, a partnership, strategically with purpose. In the *I Am Becoming Tour* across the nation, Mrs. Obama shared her authentic self to thousands of audience members explaining the importance of attitude and not being afraid to seek help when needed.

Who can help you in your purpose? What is his name? What is her name? If you have a desire to invest in real estate and it brings you joy, could your life partner be a real estate agent? What if your joy revealed was false, you may have felt it brought you joy because you made a lot of money, then your true purpose was revealed to you at a later time. You open a micro-loan business in Zimbabwe to help families start businesses. Your partner may not want to live in Zimbabwe, so you compromise to another location where you can still live life with purpose and remain at peace with your success.

Your purpose can be several things, it may seem. One ultimate purpose with several passions perhaps. When trying to identify your passions or your ultimate purpose, surround yourself around people living with purpose, continue with positive affirmations, and keep toxins away (remember they can come in the form of people).

Toxins, according to the Merriam-Webster dictionary, are poisonous substances, especially one that is produced by a living thing. Let's remove the toxins, whatever or whomever they are, and keep positive things around us to ensure we are really living our best life, strategically.

How can you keep a positive attitude?

1. Positive Affirmations you can begin with daily:

_____

_____

_____

_____

_____

_____

2. What are some toxins you need to remove?

_____

_____

_____

_____

"Find something you love to do and you'll never have to work a day in your life." ~ Harvey Mackay

Chapter **5**

Loving and Living Your Life

I wonder how many times I'd stood in line next to someone who felt pain like I had felt. I was oblivious to others' pain until it became my own. It was Mothers' Day and I had taken the day off work because it was too much to bear: people telling me "Happy Mothers' Day", assuming I was a mother at 20 years of age or assuming it was happy. Others, sharing what they would do for their mothers and how much joy it would bring them. I did not love my life because I was not living with purpose then. Several Mothers' Days into my purpose, and I now give Keynote Talks for Mothers' Day brunches.

Build a life you don't need a vacation from. We have heard this saying before. Some strive to make this a reality, while others may feel it will never be their reality. None of us leave this world alive so live it with purpose every day. Your life is not a game... but you must learn how to play the game of life if you so choose to do so. The corporate game. The military game. The political game. The public sector game. Once you know the rules of the game, you can play well. And even in this game, you must be innovative because the rules may change, the game can change, the academic game, the athletic game. Are you competitive enough to learn more? To keep growing? To keep winning? What if you do not have the same values of the rule makers? Will you still play? Will you become the change agent and make your own rules to help the greater good?

We all know at least one person like this: they wake up, complain all day, hate their job, and wait for Friday to come! Hate Mondays! Really live life on the weekends, trying to love the life they live. The others you meet, living the life they love, a purpose filled life, a life of joy daily, a life they do not need a vacation from. Golf at 11:00am on a Tuesday. Aruba on a Wednesday, fly back when you've soaked up enough sun, if you desire.

What if you could have your cake and eat it too. Really?! I mean, if you could live with purpose and have joy every day, would you trade it in for the life you currently have now? Smile more... help others more, altruistically. Trade a selfish life in for a selfless life. *The more we get, give. The more we learn, teach.* Maya Angelou reminds us of purpose strategies. Oprah Winfrey shared with the world her journey to open a school for girls in South Africa after a conversation with Nelson Mandela. I went to visit Soweto where the Nelson Mandela National Museum is located, commonly referred to as Mandela House, is the house on Vilakazi Street, Orlando West, Soweto, South Africa, where Nelson Mandela once lived. I was searching for a new location of where my work would continue to help families impacted by cancer and decrease generational poverty as well as situational poverty.

Generational poverty, passed on from generation to generation. Situation poverty can occur after someone in the household is impacted by such a disease like breast cancer. If there is only one parent in the home and income is affected due to the horrible disease, situational poverty can last for several months or even several years. Many of the families I was blessed to help, unfortunately had incidences of generational poverty combined with situational poverty where families with single head of households with an average of 2 -3 dependents were trying to survive cancer while living below the federal poverty line. The federal poverty line is based on household size. Living in Alaska and Hawaii are in different categories than the other 48 states in America because the cost of living is higher. For example, according to the Poverty Level Guidelines Chart (2019), the poverty level for a household of four is an annual income of $25,750. To get the poverty level for larger families, add $4,420 for each additional person in the household and for smaller families, subtract $4,420 per person. This number is different for Alaska and Hawaii.

Living paycheck to paycheck, as hard as it is, is made worse by being diagnosed with a disease on top of that. Then imagine your partner walks out on you, and your once trusted gainful employer walks out on you as well. Whatever happened to "till death do us part, through sickness and health?" You may or may not have a desire to be married or you may already be married. A passion could be to become married or stay married. A desire in that passion could be to have children or more children. Yes, your partner or children can bring you joy, but your purpose, that brings you ultimate joy, the ultimate climax.

Now this is different for women and men, who are stay at home moms/dads. Some have a desire that can turn into an ultimate passion or purpose if the supporting role is to be a team player so their partner could live in their ultimate purpose. Some are able to live in this role and remain content. Others feel a void or emptiness, and when that void grows, they need to have their ultimate purpose fulfilled too. They may not want to feel selfish and may not know how to share this new growth but may show you through subtle ways. Effective communication is key through these processes.

Those in relationships who fail to do so lead to divorce too often.

When I studied communication across the lifespan, I realized something so important: lifespans can be short or long for others. Lots of things can change in a lifetime. Ideas change and sometimes even beliefs and values change. I have an uncle who changed his religion to become a Muslim while still married to his wife, my Aunt, a Baptist Christian woman. They are still married and respect one another, which is very hard to do. Passions and desires can change. Which then also let us know that purpose can also change.

Your purpose as a teacher in your twenties can change from elementary grade students to going back to school and obtaining a Ph.D. to become a professor at a university. Growth is great, if that is what you desire. As long as those desires come from you and not forced because of someone else. Resentment can occur and a life of unhappiness may come with it. Perhaps your ultimate desire was always to become a professor but your passion or desire to become a teacher was the first seed planted. You were maybe unaware of your full potential; your true climactic moment occurred as a professor. Your pursuit of happiness revealed. Success!

My mother was a teacher, poet, painter, dancer, pianist, seamstress, storyteller, singer... she definitely had many passions. Her ultimate purpose, simply stated, was being an artist. Artists have many creative forms of expression. She happened to encompass all of them. Through her art, she was able to become a better teacher to reach children at various levels by being innovative in and outside the classroom.

Loving the Life You Live or ... Living the Life You Love? Do you love your life, right now?

1. Yes, I love....

_____

_____

_____

_____

_____

2. I would like to change....

_____

_____

_____

_____

_____

_____

"In any moment of decision, the best thing you can do is the right thing. The next best thing is the wrong thing, and the worst thing you can do is nothing."

~ Theodore Roosevelt

Chapter **6**

Mission: Taking Action

Do you ever feel stuck? Is it hard to act on decisions you made several weeks ago, months ago, how about years ago? I am going to help you get out of your own way by sharing some insight with you, so you can *do something.*

Here are a few common quotes to begin with. Feel free to take one that screams at you. Yes, screams at you. It can't purr at you like a little kitten, I need it to SCREAM or even ROAR at you like a lion. My recommendation would be to type it up when you are at home today and paste it on your forehead. Or perhaps by the mirror in your bathroom so you read it aloud every morning until you do something about whatever it is you are not satisfied with in your life.

1. "Just because I am struggling does NOT mean I am failing. Every great success requires some kind of struggle to get there."

2. "*Finished last* will always be better than *did not finish*, which always trumps, *did not start*."

3. "If I truly want to change my life, I must first... change my mind."

4. "Most great things in my life won't happen by chance, they will happen... by choice."

I often meet people who do nothing. They do nothing about their marriage that is falling apart, nothing about their children's failing grades, nothing about their career they hate to be in, nothing about their high blood pressure increasing, and nothing about their debt as it continues to pile higher and higher, month after month, yet wish to buy a home.

I paid off all my debt in order to buy my first house. I went back to college to complete a graduate degree to boost my education. I started a nonprofit organization with a mission to provide prevention education, economic support, and health and wellness services because I lost my mom to breast cancer. At that very moment, I knew that writing down my favorite quote really helped me do something by taking action and planning strategically. That quote was empowering to me and I posted it everywhere to read daily - **"be the change you wish to see in the world."**

By starting that nonprofit organization, I believed that I became that change. I did something. We must do something if we are unhappy about the current circumstances of our lives. We must get up and take steps to change where we are in order to do better. We must take action.

Now change doesn't happen overnight. It is even harder for someone to change if they do not see the need for change. Here are five easy steps to help you do something to create positive change in your life.

Step 1: Plan (acknowledge that change is needed, and begin to plan ways to change by brainstorming ideas)

Step 2: Organize (after you brainstorm and create your pros and cons of each idea, focus on the top 2 or 3 ideas with the most positive pros to help you change)

Step 3: Reward (give yourself a pat on the back for getting this far, as an example, if you are trying to lose weight and plan one is in action and you have already lost five pounds of 15, treat yourself, eat that pancake for breakfast with tons of syrup, eat that pizza for lunch, and eat that slice of cheesecake you wanted with your dinner. Reward yourself maybe once a week or once every two weeks and keep going with an extra boost of commitment to achieve your goals.) If you move forward accomplishing your goals and do not give yourself a reward, there is a higher chance of binging or maxing out that credit card again. Once you reward yourself, eating oatmeal six days a week for breakfast doesn't seem as bad anymore because you have something to look forward to on that Saturday morning. I absolutely love cheat days, yes #foodie.

Step 4: Manage (Now you have a good schedule going. As an example, you created an additional savings account for your next trip out of the country and each paycheck you put away is an additional $200 dollars. It is a sacrifice, meaning you will not be able to spend that extra $100 on wine every two weeks, but it is okay, you have managed a schedule and you are on your way to going on that first trip to the Virgin Islands.)

Step 5: Change (you did it!) you changed... all because you did something about it. You paid off that last credit card, you saved enough for that all-inclusive trip, you graduated with your doctorate and got promoted way above your peers, you opened up that business you always wanted to, you put away an extra $5,000.00 a year for your retirement, you reached a new level of accomplishment in your membership club.

I hope you wrote down a motivational quote that screamed at you in this book. I hope that you can apply these simple five steps to bring that change into your life. Step 1: Plan, Step 2: Organize, Step 3: Reward, Step 4: Manage, and Step 5: Change.

You deserve it! After all, you are the only one that can do something about it.

Start by doing what is possible and suddenly you are doing the impossible. Your goals are possible... all because you started by doing something.

Give me a reason to anticipate the seasons that we can reach. It is in our destination to carry on to another dimension, so walk with me. We must feel it in our spines to do something. I mean feel it to the tip of infinite possibilities that lie in the tiny particles of dust on your shoulders. Remove the boulders and chips and dust the shoulders off. Yes, you can! I believe in you. But surely, my belief is nothing without you taking action. With no action it is simply the talk without the walk. Let's add them together.

It is time to do something!

1. I will start doing ...?

_____

_____

_____

_____

_____

_____

2. I will stop doing...? Sometimes this list can be more
    important than our start list.

_____

_____

_____

_____

_____

_____

"Education is the most powerful weapon we can use to change the world."

~ Nelson Mandela

Chapter 7

Education: Values to Destiny

My mother was a teacher. Many of the youth in our village of Sion Farm, St. Croix, Virgin Islands, would come over to be taught by my mother. When she was diagnosed with breast cancer, she turned more to theatre, dance, and singing to help her (and still help others) while she battled the horrible disease. She often recited her poetry in a poetry group with Audre Lorde, who also lost the fight to breast cancer.

I read an incredible book about Audre Lorde in my Rhetoric course during my undergraduate degree at Georgia State University. Audre Lorde's book, Sister Outsider, shares evidence that both the individual and the community are valued. Audre believed the community "allows the I to be." Dr. Darsey, my former Professor, taught a great course that I am forever thankful for. I was not always a student in the top of the class until I found my niche. Courses in speech, communications, and theatre, helped me relate to my mother, the community (the village), and myself. I saw the importance of values and only then, did I begin to see the value of education, like never before. Purpose, strategically allowing the seed to grow.

In my Theatre courses, Dr. Holmes was my Professor and an incredible mentor, often reminding me of my mother's free spirit. I grew the desire to share these positive attributes on to a group of students in a program called Soldiers to Scholars based in Orlando, Florida and founded by the incredible Dr. Reddick. Soldiers to Scholars helped create an incredible mentorship program with military veteran mentees and at-risks grade school students in a disadvantaged population. I became a mentor during my graduate degree at the University of Central Florida (Go Knights!) and connected with each and every one of those students by sharing the importance of values, theatre, education, mentorship, and history.

In life, it does not matter how much education we have, how much money we have, or how much we accomplished for ourselves. It really matters how much we give back and how much we help others. The late great boxer, Muhammad Ali shares, "service to others is the rent you pay for your room here on earth." Muhammad Ali was a man of the community and a man of great values.

"Your beliefs become your thoughts,
Your thoughts become your words,
Your words become your actions,
Your actions become your habits,
Your habits become your values,
Your values become your destiny."

~ Mahatma Gandhi

While I was coaching students at the University of Central Florida out of the Office of Integrity and Ethical Development as a Certified Professional Life Coach, I always started with the importance of values when it comes to the decision-making process. We have to be aware of the choices we make in life. We are ultimately in control of our destiny. What are your values?

The seven core Army values consist of the acronym LDRSHIP.

- Loyalty – Bearing true faith and allegiance is a matter of believing in and devoting yourself to something or someone.
- Duty – Fulfill your obligations.
- Respect – Treat people as they should be treated.
- Selfless Service – Put the welfare of the nation, the Army and your subordinates before your own.
- Honor – Live up to Army values.
- Integrity – Do what is right, legally and morally.
- Personal Courage – Face fear, danger or adversity.

The three values of nonprofit organization, I Will Survive, Incorporated is the acronym IWS.

1. Innovation – Keeping good values at the forefront while completing the mission (service, integrity, transparency, inclusion, diversity, accountability).
2. Wellness – Lead by example holistically and remember health is the greatest wealth.
3. Sustainability – Create a culture of health with the people and earth in mind (reduce the generational poverty cycle).

If you do not have your own values, analyze a few companies you admire and/or people and see if there are some values that you could bring into your life. Write those values down. Become familiar with them, as you may use them subconsciously in your next Ted Talks.

Building the Foundation.

What are your values?

_____

_____

_____

_____

_____

_____

_____

Why are these values important to you?

_____

_____

_____

_____

_____

Values List

Authenticity

Achievement

Adventure

Authority

Autonomy

Balance

Beauty

Boldness

Compassion

Challenge

Community

Competency

Contribution

Creativity

Curiosity

Determination

Fairness

Faith

Friendship

Fun

Growth

Happiness

Honesty

Humor

Influence

Inner Harmony

Justice

Kindness

Knowledge

Leadership

Learning

Love

Loyalty

Meaningful Work

Openness

Optimism

Peace

Pleasure

Poise

Recognition

Religion

Reputation

Respect

Responsibility

Security

Self-Respect

Service

Spirituality

Stability

Success

Status

Trustworthiness

Wealth

Wisdom

"*Time and health are two precious assets that we don't recognize and appreciate until they have been depleted.*"

~ Denis Waitley

Chapter **8**

Self - Care with Purpose

I was in Winter Park, Florida, near Orlando. It was Thursday afternoon around 3:00pm. It was so cold, dark, lonely, as I lay there on the floor with major pain in the mid-section of my body. I could not identify where it was coming from. I managed to crawl to my phone and call for help. I called a tele-nurse through the Veterans Hospital. The pain was excruciating; it felt as if I were being stabbed. I was completing a master's program in Florida at the time, leading an organization I founded in Georgia, and juggling a few other tasks on my plate as well. I would often leave class on a Thursday night with my vehicle packed ready to drive six hours up to Georgia to host a fundraising event and visit breast cancer patients in the hospital who had no family to visit them.

I was rushed to the hospital that day and spent a few days as an in-patient myself. Lyft got me there safe and sound as I was unable to drive, the pain was that unbearable. I did not know if it was my heart, my lungs. But I felt my mid-section suffering. Several tests were run in order to identify where these major pains came from inside of my body. I was blessed to have visitors and so thankful to this day, the little things remembering the ladies I would visit who has no visitors while they were in the hospital for surgery or treatments for breast cancer. My doctor came back the last of the three days I was there, being still and informing me that I would be released soon and that I suffered from acute pancreatitis. He said I needed to take better care of myself. Stress almost killed me while I was living a purposeful life. I went through a major detox. Planned ways to incorporate more stress relief tactics. Asked for help more, delegated more instead of trying to do it all by myself. I then worked on getting my for-profit business a little more on auto pilot. Lastly, I created some principles and took out my calendar to schedule some Anisa time. If I did not schedule it, it did not happen.

The organization I ran went from being open 24/7, to 3 days a week to the public. We had a strict 24 hour turn around rate to thank donors once the organization had received donations as well as clients reaching out to us in need of support. My staff was small, volunteer-run, mostly. I scheduled time to workout more and bought a new bike. I was able to schedule time to travel more, read more, relax more, and spend more time with family. I moved further away from the city when moving back to Georgia. I bought my first home and breathed. More Anisa time mattered for me. Do not end up in the hospital to realize this for yourself. Stress can kill.

I want to share six principles that have helped me over the last few years since my emergency scare. You can come up with your own principles but before you do, try this APP out. It is the Anisa Palmer Principles™ to living your life with purpose. Once you download these into your life, you will begin to see a change in your lifestyle and perhaps, even your values. These will also help so you do not get burnt out while living your purposeful life.

- Principle 1: **Travel Much**
- Principle 2: **Laugh Daily**
- Principle 3: **Chew Slowly**
- Principle 4: **Dance Often**
- Principle 5: **Sing Aloud**
- Principle 6: **Love Self**

"The more you read, the more things you will know. The more that you learn, the more places you will go." Dr. Seuss encouraged me to go more places along with my incredible Aunt, my father's twin sister, Denise, whom I often called Mama Gayla. Mama Gayla has been to all the continents on this earth except Antarctica and has no desire to go there. The late phenomenal woman, Maya Angelou, also reminds us to "travel to as many destinations as possible for the sake of education as well as pleasure." I learned so much while traveling to South Africa, Cuba, Aruba, Spain, France, Barbados, Italy, Jamaica, and many more. The culture in all these places are very unique along with the food, music, people. I often enjoyed becoming a #foodie in these places and decided to write "travel" into my annual business and personal plans even more. Why? Sometimes, if we do not plan, it does not happen right?! In the military, we often used the 5 P's: Proper Planning Prevents Poor Performance. Another common one is from Benjamin Franklin — "If you fail to plan, you are planning to fail!"

When I became an entrepreneur again, I realized that if it was not in my calendar, planned, I would not go on vacation and take time for self. Hence, travel much became the 1st principle to live a more purpose filled life. The 2nd principle, was planted while serving in the military, when a fellow battle buddy came to me and said, "you are always so serious, do you ever laugh?" I got really good at separating my professional and personal life. I was silly with family and close friends; however, military life was really 24/7 for active duty personnel. I didn't know how to separate it anymore and I began to turn all emotions off to never allow anyone to see the soft caring side of Sergeant Palmer. My dear sister really woke me up when I saw her cry because of something I said to unintentionally offend her. She was not pregnant nor on her menstrual cycle. I had to dig deep and see who I was becoming and what I said that would bring those tears from her beautiful eyes to fall on her lovely brown cheeks. I needed more laughter in my life. I needed to laugh daily.

Daily laughter heals the soul. We should race to get these laughs in daily. Find a laughter yoga class and join it if you see yourself in where I used to be. This is very unhealthy. If you would like to study some of the research out there on humor and laughter, Professor Rod Martin or Dr. Martin's research interests me and may interest you as well. His research began in 1980 as a Professor of clinical psychology at the University of Western Ontario. Additional research you may find interesting is from the Journal of Epidemiology, where laughter was studied for ameliorating symptoms of depression, dementia, and insomnia. I suffered from two of three of these conditions while serving in the military during combat in Iraq.

Principle 3, came from standing in a mess hall line to get food as military personnel, especially in boot camp. You may only have a few minutes to eat in your allotted time or you may not get a chance to eat at all, so the goal was to shove as much food as you can into your mouth. If you needed to use the restroom, this also took away from "food devouring" time and certainly no time for #foodie pictures on Instagram. I kept the horrible habit of devouring my food and never took the time to enjoy it while serving in the Armed Forces and even kept this up a year or two after I received an honorable discharge and separated from the military. Studies show us that eating slowly contributes to a lower risk of obesity for normal weight, overweight, and obese adults. When we eat slowly, we can actually pay attention to what we are putting in our mouth. Have you ever eaten something and not known what is was? But why?

If you noticed, all of these principles cover our human needs with a holistic approach, similar to Maslow's hierarchy of needs. We need food, but when chewed slowly, as in principle 3, we can reach self-actualization and increased self-esteem.

In principle 4, dance often came to me as an exercise. Dancing is an exercise, and in the 2000's we saw an increase of dance routines incorporated in workouts at gyms and separate dance studios opened all over various cities, particularly, Atlanta. We needed to find innovative ways to get people active and even new stripper imitated dance classes were born, pole fitness dance classes.

Caribbean people dance year-round at carnivals with or without music. I saw that I was missing a piece of dance in my life. Someone, so rudely, turned off the music that often played in my head and I stopped dancing. I had to get the music back on. Running and dancing both boosted my metabolism, kept my heart healthy so I didn't have to see Cardiologist and TV

Personality, Dr. David Montgomery at PreVent Clinic, both released positive endorphins, gave me sexy calf muscles and gave me the necessary cardio recommended for an adult. Even people with two left feet have a blast dancing. Dance as if no one is watching and see how great it feels. Get a full dance in to your favorite song using your full body. And no... car dancing jam out sessions do not count! P. Diddy, musical legend, even challenged Atlanta recently to encourage more peaches and peach implants to dance at dance clubs, no more posting up on a wall.

Similar to principle 4, principle 5 can be done when no one is listening. When was the last time you sang aloud? Maybe in the car stuck in traffic with ongoing drivers looking at you like you are crazy as if they somehow can't hear the incredible music jamming through your speakers. Maybe you are shy and choose not to share your voice with others so you hold back on being ultimately free and living your life unapologetically. Release... it will make you feel that much better, in addition to more health benefits. Ask a singer about it.

Now you have all the tools needed to find your purpose ... and not let it kill you. When it is revealed to you, you can be ready. You will know how to act. You can live a purposeful life. Say YES to you. When you do, you also say yes to others around you and begin to live a life bigger than you.

Placing the Puzzle Together.

My life principles are...?

_____

_____

_____

_____

_____

_____

_____

_____

_____

_____

_____

_____

_____

_____

My passions are...?

_____

_____

_____

_____

_____

_____

_____

_____

_____

_____

My purpose is...?

_____

_____

_____

_____

My **Self Care Methods** will include ...

_____

_____

_____

_____

_____

_____

_____

_____

_____

_____

_____

About the Author

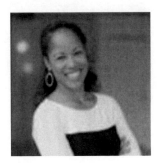

Anisa Palmer, a St. Croix, Virgin Islands native, was a combat veteran of the Army and currently resides in Georgia. Anisa has a Bachelor's of Arts in Speech - Communications from Georgia State University, a Master's in Public Administration from the University of Central Florida, is a Certified Professional Life Coach, a proud Junior League of Atlanta member and a Certified Nonprofit Professional. Anisa lives a life of service through various philanthropic efforts and is the CEO of the Palmer Firm Group, LLC. As a fond member of the Georgia, Florida and the Caribbean communities, Anisa prides herself on being a good human being, Forbes Contributor, United States Virgin Islands Tourism Ambassador, Health Advocate, Mentor, Author, Public Speaker and Purpose Strategist.

Stay Connected.

AnisaPalmer.com
IG @OfficialAnisaPalmer
Facebook @PalmerFirmGroup
#TheUtlimateClimax #PurposeStrategist

IWillSurviveInc.org
IG, Facebook, Twitter @IWillSurviveInc